Essential Living

Aromatherapy Recipes
for Health & Home

2nd Edition
Copyright © 2015 Andrea Butje
All rights reserved.
ISBN-10: 1477533338
ISBN-13: 978-1477533338

For my Cindy

Sitting quietly

Continuing to be

The most inspiring person I know

I love being on this journey with you!

Your Andrea

Acknowledgments:

Recipe for Essential Living

Makes: One book

Ingredients:
1 oz (30 ml) Cindy Black (www.bigtreehealing.com)
1 oz (30 ml) Andi Graham (www.bigseadesign.com)
1 oz (30 ml) Laura Irmis (www.laurairmis.com)
1 oz (30 ml) Maria Mora (www.mariamora.info)
1 oz (30 ml) Annette Scott (hattie@hattieppink.com)
100 drops Aromahead Institute Students and Graduates

Tools:
Computer
Caffeine
A Kitchen

Directions:
Use the Stovetop Melting Method to combine your inspiration with organization. Ask Maria and Annette to write, edit and stir, have Andi and Laura create beautiful designs and test every recipe with the Aromahead students and graduates. Be sure to have Cindy make you laugh out loud every day!

Notes:
It's always a good idea to have people you love and admire contribute their extraordinary skills.

Contents:

Chapter I Introduction to Aromatherapy

Aromatherapy: It's Surprisingly Scientific!
Aromatherapy isn't a mystical, new age concept. It's grounded in science and chemistry. (Don't worry; you won't need to learn any chemistry to use Aromatherapy in your everyday routines.)

Aromatherapy is all about the therapeutic use of essential oils—highly aromatic substances that occur naturally in plants. Essential oils are made up of naturally occurring chemical components that have all sorts of therapeutic properties. Through decades of research, scientists have identified hundreds of these chemical components and learned what they do. Some are antibacterial, some are sedative, and some are antispasmodic. These chemical components contribute to the overall effects of essential oils.

Essential oils also affect people on emotional levels that can be harder to define through research. This is where the brain and sense of smell come in to play. We know that lavender essential oil has properties that calm the body—but we also know that the smell alone can be emotionally comforting and calming.

Don't like lavender? Individuals react to smells in many different ways; don't worry if you don't feel the way you "should" when you smell certain oils. When making your own products, always feel free to skip oils you're not fond of.

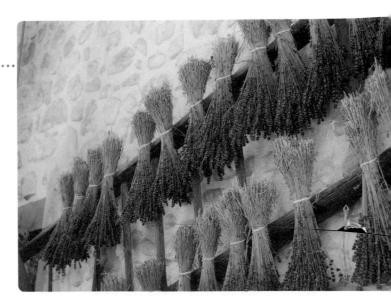

Bouquets of lavender drying in France.

Plants: The Foundation of Aromatherapy

Have you ever cleaned your hands with a fresh slice of lemon? Have you ever cooked with a fresh sprig of rosemary or used dried herbs in a sachet of potpourri? If so, you were experiencing a preview of the power of essential oils.

While Aromatherapists use a wide variety of natural oils and butters to create therapeutic products, they can't practice Aromatherapy without pure essential oils distilled from plants. Essential oils are extracted from different parts of plants, including flowers, fruit rinds, seeds, leaves and even roots. Distillers extract essential oil from large quantities of plant material.

People have understood the healing power of plants for centuries. Herbal medicine and flower remedies are two other forms of alternative medicine that involve plant-based healing.

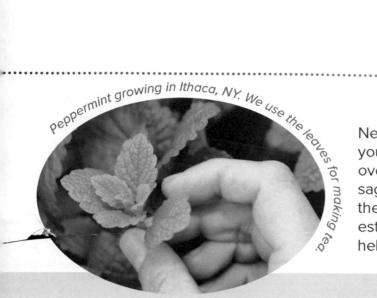

Peppermint growing in Ithaca, NY. We use the leaves for making tea.

Next time you're in your garden or browsing through your local nursery, take a moment to run your fingers over the leaves of aromatic plants like peppermint, sage and thyme. The scent left on your fingers is from the plant's essential oils. Many beginners find that establishing a connection with aromatic plants can help develop intuitive Aromatherapy blending skills.

Beware Impostors: Synthetic Fragrances

Essential oils can't be created synthetically. They only occur in nature.

Check out the labels of some of the bath and body care products you have around the house. If you see the word, "parfum" or "fragrance," the aroma of the product comes from chemicals (synthetic fragrances), not essential oils. Studies have shown that synthetic fragrances are often irritating to the skin. In some cases synthetics and chemicals may cause other health concerns. If you have skin sensitivities or allergies, it's especially important to consider avoiding synthetic fragrances.

Aromatherapy should not be confused with scented products. Often, major consumer brands market everything from candles to dish soap as Aromatherapy products. This is just clever marketing. Learn to read labels when you're shopping for products that you don't make at home.

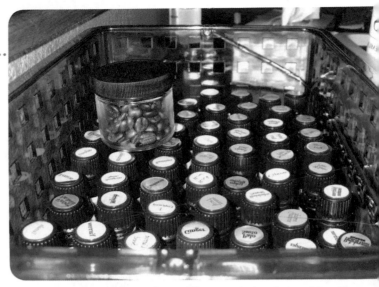

Aromatherapy is beginner friendly.

Is Aromatherapy Beginner Friendly?

Yes. Clinical Aromatherapists formulate special blends for many ailments and purposes. Essential oil blends and salves can be used to soothe pain and inflammation, to help with menstrual cramps, and to encourage scar healing. In order to blend at this level of expertise, Aromatherapists study essential oil safety, human anatomy, and basic chemistry. In the United States, the National Association for Holistic Aromatherapy and the Alliance of International Aromatherapists set strict education standards and guidelines for best practices.

However, as a beginner, you don't need a certification to use essential oils around the home. All you need are the right tools and safety guidelines. Dilution guidelines exist to ensure that your Aromatherapy products are safe and gentle.

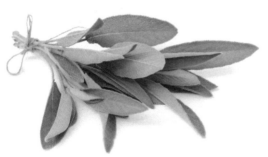

After putting together a basic Aromatherapy tool kit, you can begin creating body butters, Aromatherapy sprays, inhalers, cleaning products and more. Experiment with aromas and you'll quickly learn what you love and what works for you and your family. As your skills become more advanced, you may find yourself inspired to learn more about the art and chemistry of Aromatherapy.

Chapter 2 Your Essential Oil Toolkit

Getting Started with the Blending Basics

Every Aromatherapist has a collection of essential oils. You don't need dozens of oils to begin. When you're just getting started, add to your collection slowly. As you blend, you'll discover the oils you love the most, and the carriers and tools you use most often.

Buying Essential Oils

Give yourself a budget and adjust it according to how often you blend and the types of blends you use. Some oils will last you five or six years; others will be used up within a year.

Because of the amount of material used and the amount of effort put in to growing and harvesting the plant material, many essential oils can be expensive. Beware of inexpensive oils—these are often synthetic or cut with adulterants. Perfume oils and synthetic essential oils aren't effective and can oftentimes cause skin irritation and allergic reactions. As a general rule, you should be wary of essential oils you find at grocery stores and markets, especially if they're all the same price.

The real workhorses—like tea tree, lemon and lavender—are very affordable.

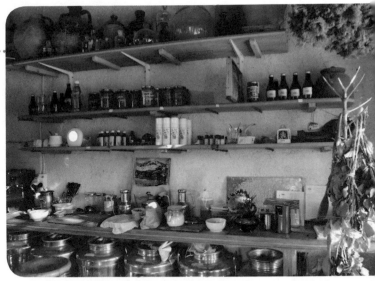

Kitchen at the Wild Herbs of Crete in Greece.

Buy larger sizes when you can; they're generally more cost effective this way. When it comes to pricier oils, try a few from different aromatic families. Consider a good base note and a good floral.

How to Store and Care for Your Oils

This is easy! Here is the trick to maintaining the vitality of your essential oils: Store them in a closed, dark glass container, out of the sun, in a cool place.

Simply stated, keep the caps on your oils when you are finished using them and store them in a refrigerator or cool closet. Oxygen, sunlight and heat speed up oxidation (the process which breaks down your essential oils). When essential oils are stored cold their shelf lives improve.

Essential oil shelf life varies. The storage conditions make a significant difference. Ask the company you buy your oils from to provide you with the shelf life for each oil you purchase and then make a note of when you need to replace each one.

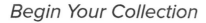

Begin Your Collection

A good starter kit would include:

Eucalyptus globulus *(Eucalyptus globulus)*

Frankincense *(Boswellia carterii)*

Grapefruit *(Citrus paradisi)*

Lavender *(Lavandula angustifolia)*

Lemon *(Citrus limon)*

Lemongrass *(Cymbopogon citratus)*

Orange *(Citrus sinensis)*

Palmarosa *(Cymbopogon martini var. motia)*

Peppermint *(Mentha x piperita)*

Rosemary ct. Camphor *(Rosmarinus officinalis ct camphor/1,8 cineole)*

Tea Tree *(Melaleuca alternifolia)*

White Pine *(Pinus strobus)*

These are some great oils to add as you increase your collection:

Cypress *(Cupressus sempervirens)*

Geranium *(Pelargonium roseum x asperum)*

Juniper *(Juniperus communis)*

Distilled Lime *(Citrus aurantifolia)*

Mandarin *(Citrus reticulata)*

Ravintsara *(Cinnamomum camphora ct 1,8 cineole)*

Roman Chamomile *(Chamaemelum nobile)*

Siberian Fir *(Abies sibirica)*

Ylang Ylang *(Cananga odorata)*

There is a master list of all the oils used in this book in the resource section.

Buying Carrier Oils

Generally speaking, carrier oils and butters will be used directly on the skin. These are the rich, moisturizing plant extracts that make up the backbone of many Aromatherapy blends. Prices vary depending on where the plants are grown and how the carrier oils are extracted.

A good starter kit would include:

- Aloe vera gel – 8 oz (224 gm)
- Avocado oil – 8 oz (240 ml)
- Castile liquid soap – 8 oz (240 ml)
- Cocoa butter – 4 oz (112 gm)
- Coconut oil – 16 oz (448 gm)
- Hydrosols *(lavender, rose and sweetgrass)*

- Jojoba wax *(also called jojoba oil)* – 16 oz (480 ml)
- Rose hip seed oil – 4 oz (120 ml)
- Salt – 16 oz (448 gm) *(pink Himalayan or sea salts are good possibilities)*
- Shea butter – 8 oz (224 gm)
- Tamanu oil – 4 oz (120 ml)
- Trauma oil *(herbally infused oil containing Arnica, Calendula, and St. John's Wort)* – 4 oz (120 ml)
- Unscented, natural lotion – 8 oz (224 gm)
- Vitamin E oil – 1 oz (30 ml)

Additional Tools and Containers

In order to create your blends, you'll need some basic tools. You probably already have many of the tools in your kitchen. These include:

- Mixing bowls

- A kitchen scale

- A Pyrex or similar heat-safe bowl

- Stirring spoons

- Measuring cups

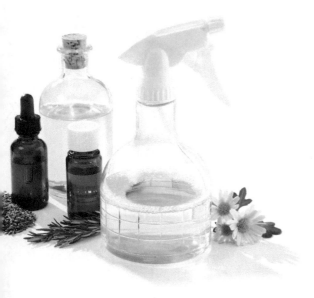

You'll need to purchase the following specialty containers for your blends:

- At least a dozen blank Aromatherapy inhalers

- Four to six glass or sturdy PET plastic stirring rods. PET plastic is known as a non-reactive plastic that doesn't leach. In cases where glass isn't ideal, PET plastic is a good choice.

- 1 oz (30 ml) glass or PET plastic bottles with lids

- 4 oz (120 ml) glass, PET plastic or aluminum spray bottles

- Several industrial-sized PET plastic spray bottles for cleaning solution

- 4 oz (120 ml) bottles and jars with lids

by Andrea Butje

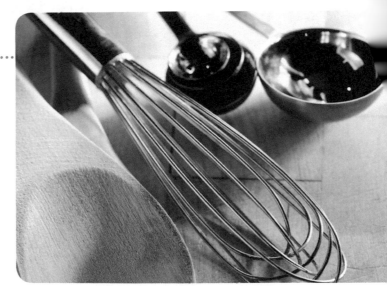

You may already have some basic tools in your home.

Many of these tools and containers can be found in craft supply stores. Once you discover what sizes and materials you prefer, try shopping online to find more variety and better deals. If you have friends who also enjoy blending, consider chipping in on bulk orders for a better price on individual units.

Purchasing Tips

- When purchasing carriers, it's absolutely crucial to make sure they haven't been refined or altered in any way.

- Watch out for fragrances or bleaching processes.

- Look for certified organic oils when possible, and check with the distributor to find out if the oils are unrefined.

- If you see chemical ingredients you don't recognize, be cautious.

- Shop online to find the best options.

Staying Organized

It's perfectly okay to start out with something as simple as a plastic box with a lid or a basket in your kitchen. Keep your supplies organized and make a point of cleaning up thoroughly after you're done blending.

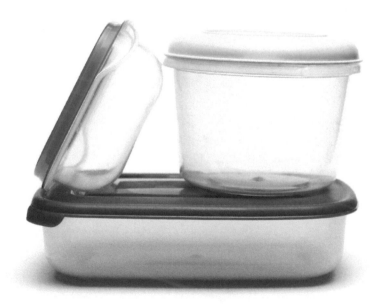

Organization Tips

- Keep all of your larger items in a big bin, preferably with a lid. This makes it easy to get everything out at once when you're ready to blend. Store your most frequently used essential oils separately, so you can access them easily. Keep all of your finished blends in a cool, dark place. To minimize heat damage, avoid leaving them out on windowsills or in your car. Store your essential oil bottles together in a plastic basket or bin with a lid so that you can transport them easily.

- Keep blends and supplies out of the reach of children and pets.

- Save your budget for the oils and carriers. Look for storage containers at discount retailers or yard sales.

- Label everything clearly, especially if you decant bulk oils and carriers into smaller containers. Always label your blends explicitly with the date you made them.

- If you begin blending for friends, consider purchasing a craft tote or hard case to bring a small kit with you. People love smelling the oils and getting a sense of different aromas and notes.

Chapter 3 Basic Aromatherapy Applications

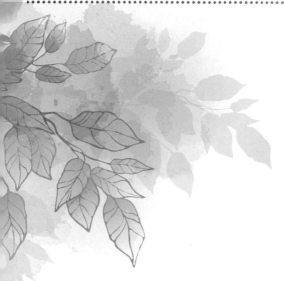

Blending Techniques

Essential oils are not generally used neat (directly from the bottle, undiluted). This means that they're diluted in different types of carriers, ranging from oils to lotions to plain water. In the previous chapter, you learned about the types of carriers you'll need to create the recipes in this book.

The methods you'll use are very simple. If you've cooked a meal, you can follow these tutorials. Most involve some careful pouring, stirring, and simple direction following.

Aromatherapists use well-researched dilution standards to ensure safety for blends used directly on the skin.

The recipes in this book follow these dilution standards:

1% Dilution: 5-6 drops per 1 oz (30 ml). Used for children between ages 5 and 12, the elderly, pregnant women and people with long-term illnesses or immune systems disorders. A 1% dilution is also a good place to start with individuals who are generally sensitive to fragrances, chemicals or other environmental pollutants.

2% Dilution: 10-12 drops per 1 oz (30 ml). Used for skin care, for natural perfumes, bath oils and for blends used frequently.

3% Dilution: 15-18 drops per 1 oz (30 ml). Used for specific, acute health concerns such as pain relief or colds and flu.

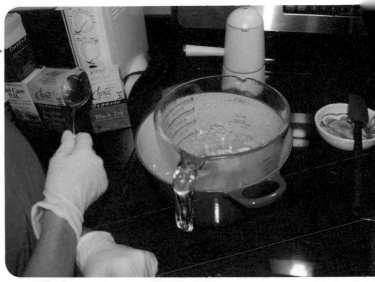

Melting body butters in class at Aromahead Institute.

The Stovetop Melting Method

To make specialized products like healing salves and lip balms, you'll need to melt a variety of ingredients together to achieve the right consistency.

We like to use what we call the Stovetop Melting Method. In recipes involving melting and pouring, we'll refer to this method. Print it out and keep it next to the stove for quick reference until you've memorized the steps. (Don't worry; it will come naturally to you quickly!)

You'll need a wide soup pan (3 quart/2.8 litre or bigger) and a 16 oz (480 ml) Pyrex measuring cup to get started. The Pyrex has to fit inside the pot. Fill the pan about 1/4 full with water, put the Pyrex cup in that pan, and use these as a double boiler. Once the water has come to a boil, lower it to a simmer and add ingredients in the following order, stirring frequently. I can tell you from personal experience that this is not the time to multi-task! Stay in front of the stove the whole time.

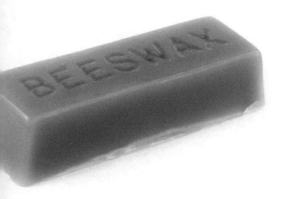

Stovetop Melting Method

- Beeswax and jojoba are first (if jojoba is applicable).
- Once beeswax and jojoba are melted, add the hardest butter.
- Once melted, add all the other hard ingredients.
- Then add softer ingredients like coconut oil.
- Leave on the heat only until melted.
- Once melted, take off the heat and add the liquid oils and shea butter and stir until melted.
- Once fully melted, add essential oils to the melted butter, stir, and pour into your jars.
- Cover the jars right away.

Tips for Working with Hot Carriers

Always be cautious when working with liquefied waxes, butters and oils. Use the same safety measures you would use when cooking hot food or oil on the stove. It's important to keep an eye on your work—don't leave hot liquids unattended. As long as you're careful (forget multi-tasking) and approach the blending as you would any type of cooking, it isn't scary!

Be sure to add the most delicate materials last—your light oils and essential oils.

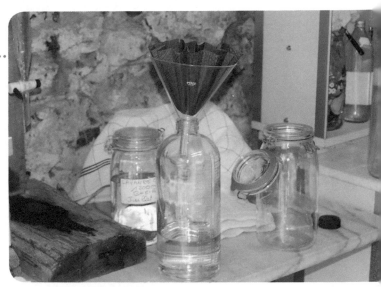

Lavender essential oil being filtered after distillation.

Workspace and Cleanup

Wondering where to blend? All you really need is some countertop space. Work with what you have. This might be a desk in your craft room, your kitchen counter next to the sink, or your dining room table.

Dish washing liquid is all you need to clean up oil and carrier residue. If you're working on a surface that stains, consider using a surface protector. Kitchen supply stores carry silicon mats that make great surfaces to work on if you're concerned with spills.

Be sure to thoroughly clean up when you're done to avoid oily surfaces. Try using a few paper towels to wipe off any excess carrier oil or butter before washing with soap and water. This makes clean up much easier. Also take care to minimize exposure of your carriers and oils to air. Check every lid to make sure the caps are screwed on tight. If you keep your workspace clean and your process smooth, you'll have more fun blending.

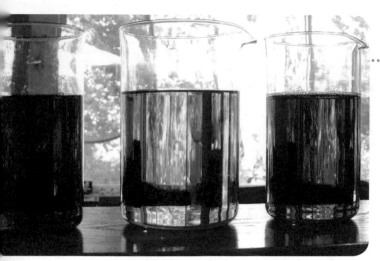

Orange, bergamot and pink grapefruit essential oils.

Free Form Blending

The Drop-by-Drop Blending Technique

While Aromatherapists often use tried and true recipes, they also create their own unique blends, using a variety of techniques to address specific concerns and intentions. As you develop your skills, take time to learn more about each essential oil with which you work. You may start to become comfortable tweaking blends—especially to change a blend's aroma to suit your personal preferences. When blending in this manner, always use the Drop-By-Drop Blending Technique, detailed here.

- Arrange your collection of oils at your workspace.
  (We like to keep them all in a convenient plastic bin with handles.)
- Choose two to six oils you'd like to work with.
- Use a notepad to track your progress.
- Add one drop of an essential oil to your carrier first. Try starting with the strongest-smelling oil.
- Add one drop of the next oil, mix, and pause to smell what these first two oils are like together.
- Continue adding one drop of each oil and pausing to smell the new aroma.
- Once you have added one of each drop, then you can begin to layer the blend by continuing to add drops of each oil to your blend.
- Once the blend smells perfect, you can stop. Just be sure not to exceed the safe dilution requirements.

Application Methods

Essential oils are generally applied on the skin in a lotion or vegetable oil (often called a carrier oil), inhaled, used in cleaning or diffused in the air. The application methods can vary widely—from a moisturizer you use at night to a spray you use to clean your kitchen counters. We'll introduce many types of application methods, which include:

Room Sprays	Jojoba Blends	Surface Sprays
Body Sprays	Lotion Blends	Surface Scrubs
Balms and Salves	Inhalers	Linen Sprays
Body Butters	Diffusers	
Moisturizers	Steam Application	

Each individual recipe in this book includes basic application instructions. As you become more familiar with the oils and carriers, you may find yourself experimenting and tweaking recipes and applications. Just remember to adhere to safety dilution guidelines. That may require a calculator.

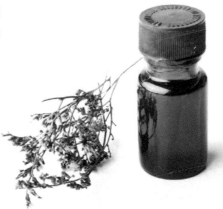

Chapter 4 The Kitchen

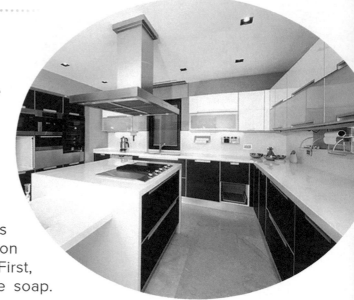

Cleaning in the Kitchen

In addition to the recipes we suggest for use in the kitchen, you can incorporate essential oils into your daily cleaning routines with some of these simple tricks.

Cutting Boards

To keep wooden and plastic cutting boards free of bacteria, use a few drops of lemon essential oil to clean the cutting board. First, wash the board with hot water and castile soap.

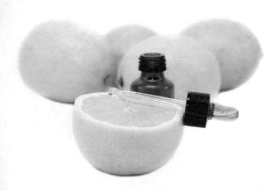

Then put about five drops of lemon essential oil on a clean sponge and wipe the board vigorously, front and back. The "side effect" is that the sponge is now also clean and bacteria free!

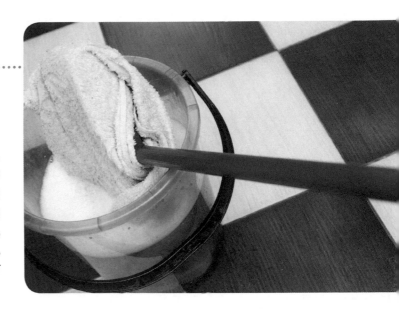

Floors

Use hydrosols and hot water on the floors. Any mop will do, but we suggest mops with a removable terry cloth cleaning surface. They're great for cleaning hardwood floors, ceramic tile, marble, and vinyl. They also work well on ceilings, walls, and windows. The terry cloth cover is removable and is machine washable.

When cleaning floors, soak the terry cloth cover (or regular mop) in hot water. Squeeze the water out and then pour a capful (a few tablespoons) of lavender hydrosol or sweetgrass hydrosol directly onto the mop.

Pets

We do not recommend using essential oils on the surfaces with which your small pets have contact.

There is some debate as to whether the essential oils on the floor would disturb the pet or have a toxic effect over time. We recommend hot water and hydrosols as a safe, effective way to clean the floors.

Recipe Difficulty Key

Beginner *

Intermediate **

Advanced ***

Directions: Simply add the drops of essential oil directly into the spray bottle full of water.

Close well, shake, and you're ready to spray.

Notes: Spray on glass surfaces, windows, kitchen counters and bathroom surfaces. I also use this spray to clean the inside of my refrigerator.

Always spot test this spray first to make sure the spray does not stain or otherwise harm your surfaces. Sometimes a surface coating will be eroded by essential oils.

Shake all spray blends each time you use them.

Surface Cleaner *
Makes: One 16 oz (480 ml) PET spray bottle
Ingredients:
15 oz (450 ml) water
1 oz (30 ml) white vinegar
20 drops Eucalyptus globulus essential oil
30 drops White Pine essential oil
30 drops Lemon essential oil
Tools:
16 oz (480 ml) PET plastic spray bottle

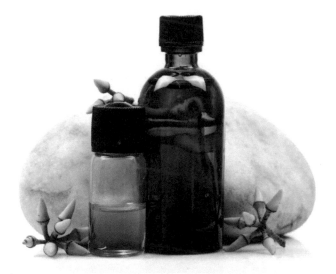

Deodorizing Spray for Trash *

Makes: One 16 oz (480 ml) spray bottle

Ingredients:

15 oz (450 ml) water

1 oz (30 ml) white vinegar

20 drops Peppermint essential oil

30 drops Orange essential oil

30 drops Lemon essential oil

Tools:

16 oz (480 ml) PET plastic spray bottle

Directions: Simply add the drops of essential oil directly into the spray bottle full of water.

Close well, shake, and you're ready to spray.

Notes: I like to spray the trashcan in my bathroom and kitchen each time I empty the trash bag. I simply take out the bag, spray the can three or four times, and add the new bag.

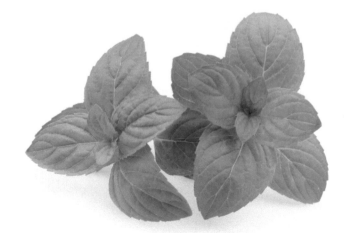

Chapter 5 The Bathroom

Making the Bathroom an Oasis

The bathroom isn't always the most pleasant-smelling room in your home. Common household cleaners use harsh chemicals to overpower smells and to disinfect. Unfortunately, these chemical cleaners aren't great for your body and can contain everything from corrosives to allergens. Who wants to take a long, luxurious bath with the smell of bleach in the air?

Chemical-Free Cleaning

Create your own antifungal cleaning spray for bathroom surfaces like tile and shower curtains. It has a bright, clean aroma without using fragrance chemicals to trick you into thinking you're smelling something clean.

The deodorizing bathroom spray can be customized to your personal preferences. We like to create different sprays throughout the year for variety and to match the season (citruses in the summer, pines for the fall, winter and holiday seasons, and florals in the spring). Use this to freshen the bathroom any time it needs a more pleasant aroma.

Our natural grout scrub uses the gentle abrasive powers of baking soda and the proven cleaning power of vinegar to get the nooks and crannies of your bathroom clean. Essential oils make this natural scrub especially effective.

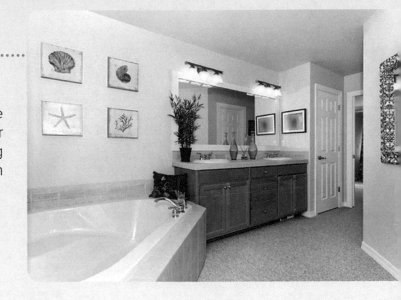

Remember, when cleaning with hand-made cleaning products, you'll need some of your own energy. Use a sturdy sponge or cleaning rag and some elbow grease to get the bathroom sparkling—naturally.

Antifungal Cleaning Spray *

Makes: One 16 oz (480 ml) spray bottle

Ingredients:

15 oz (450 ml) water

1 tablespoon white vinegar

40 drops Tea Tree essential oil

30 drops Geranium essential oil

40 drops Palmarosa essential oil

Substitution: If you don't have palmarosa, use lemon essential oil instead.

Tools:

16 oz (480 ml) PET plastic spray bottle

Directions: Fill spray bottle with 15 oz (450 ml) water.

Add the white vinegar and essential oils.

Shake vigorously before using.

Notes: Regularly spray your shower curtain and damp areas of the bath or shower liberally to prevent mold and mildew. Never use this spray on the skin. We use this spray to prevent mold on patio furniture and screened porches.

Deodorizing Bathroom Spray *

Makes: One 2 oz (60 ml) spray bottle

Ingredients:

2 oz (60 ml) water

20 drops essential oil

For a Citrus Aroma:

8 drops Grapefruit essential oil

7 drops Lemon essential oil

5 drops Orange essential oil

For a Floral Aroma:

5 drops Geranium essential oil

5 drops Jasmine absolute

10 drops Lavender essential oil

For a Pine Aroma:

20 drops White Pine essential oil

Tools:

2 oz (60 ml) spray bottle

Directions: Fill spray bottle with 2 oz (60 ml) water.

Add the essential oils.

Shake vigorously before using.

Notes: When you run out of this deodorizing air spray, use the same 2 oz (60 ml) spray bottle for each new blend—no need to use a new bottle each time.

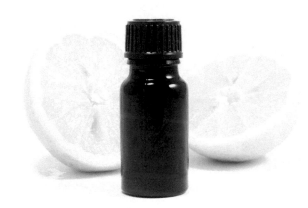

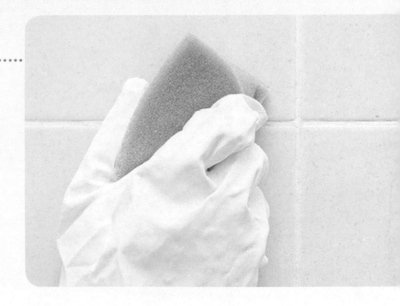

Grout Scrub **

Makes: One 8 oz (240 ml) tub of grout scrub

Ingredients:

1 cup baking soda (8 oz/224 gm)

3 tablespoons castile soap

1 tablespoon white vinegar

10 drops White Pine essential oil

10 drops Tea Tree essential oil

10 drops Lemongrass essential oil

Tools:

10 or 12 oz (300 or 360 ml) wide mouth PET plastic container/tub with fitted top. This larger container makes it easier to mix your ingredients.

Directions: Pour the 8 oz (224 gm) of baking soda into the container.

Add the castile soap and mix.

Add the white vinegar and mix (it will bubble a little).

Add all the essential oils and mix, then put the cover on.

Place a small handful of the scrub on an abrasive sponge and clean the grout.

Notes: Although essential oils are very safe, some can irritate your skin. With this blend I wear cleaning gloves.

Chapter 6 Beauty & Skin

Caring for Body and Skin

One quick trip to your local drug store or beauty department will show you how many products are marketed toward women who are trying to care for their bodies and skin. Products fight aging and wrinkles, they improve the skin tone and they moisturize or remove oil. What you may not know is that most of these products use chemicals and synthetic fragrances that can irritate your skin and pollute your body. It's important to care for your skin, especially as you age. This can be done naturally, without resorting to synthetic products.

Healthy Beauty Solutions

How do you get around fragrance chemicals and navigate the confusing ingredients listed on beauty products? If you're not a chemist, it can be near impossible to understand what you're putting on your body. Our solution? Hand-made beauty products using simple ingredients and organic sources whenever possible.

This chapter will help you create a skin care regime specific to your needs, as well as create a natural perfume balm that doesn't contain harsh synthetic fragrances. Because these products are used on your face and body—and thus close to your nose—you may require some trial and error to discover what works best for your aromatic preferences and skin type.

You may find that you use a moisturizing hydrosol during the summer months and a stronger facial moisturizer in a cream during the dry winter months. Create these products in small batches and change them up whenever needed.

Natural Deodorant ***

Makes: About six to eight .35 oz (10 ml) deodorant tubes *(depending on how high you fill them)*

Ingredients:

.5 oz (14 gm) beeswax

.5 oz (15 ml) jojoba oil

1 oz (28 gm) coconut oil

Woodsy Aroma

10 drops Cypress essential oil

5 drops distilled Lime essential oil

Floral Aroma

10 drops Geranium essential oil

5 drops Orange essential oil

Tools:

Kitchen scale

Large Pyrex measuring bowl

Medium stovetop pot

Glass stirring rod

Six to eight .35 oz (10 ml) balm/deodorant tubes

Directions: Use the Stovetop Melting Method to liquefy and combine the base carriers.

After removing the combined oils and butters from heat, add the essential oils and stir.

Immediately pour the liquid into the deodorant tubes and cover.

Allow deodorant to solidify for at least five minutes before applying.

Notes: If you prefer different aromas, feel free to create your own essential oil blend using no more than 15 total drops. Always ensure that you're using skin-nourishing oils in a deodorant blend. Because this deodorant contains no harsh chemicals or antiperspirant, you may need to apply a few times a day.

Soothing Salt Scrub *

Makes: One 4 oz (120 ml) jar of salt scrub

Ingredients:

2 oz (56 gm) salt

(I like pink Himalayan salt or sea salt)

1 oz (30 ml) jojoba oil

5 drops Grapefruit essential oil

10 drops Frankincense essential oil

Tools:

One 4 oz (120 ml) PET plastic jar

Stirring spoon

Directions: Combine the salt and carrier oil directly in the PET plastic jar.

Add the drops of essential oils and stir vigorously with a spoon.

Notes: Use a small handful while you're in the shower or bath to scrub away dead skin and soothe muscle aches. Avoid use on the face. Rinse well. The lingering layer of jojoba will provide long lasting moisture.

This blend is wonderful for soothing sore muscles after a workout. For a silkier texture and sweet aroma, try adding a teaspoon of coconut oil to this recipe.

Restorative Moisturizer *

Makes: One 2 oz (60 ml) jar of moisturizer for the face

Ingredients:

2 oz (56 gm) organic unscented lotion

10 drops Carrot Seed essential oil

5 drops Neroli essential oil

Tools:

2 oz (60 ml) glass or PET plastic jar with a lid

Glass stirring rod

Directions: Fill empty jar with unscented lotion.

Add drops directly to lotion and stir for at least one minute.

Notes: It is always a good idea to test a facial blend on the inside of your wrist for a few hours to check for skin sensitivities. Apply to freshly cleaned skin at morning and night. Feel free to add one or two more drops of either oil if you prefer a stronger aroma.

Dry Skin Moisturizer *

Makes: One 2 oz (60 ml) jar of moisturizer for the face

Ingredients:

2 oz (56 gm) organic unscented lotion

10 drops Sandalwood essential oil

10 drops Lavender essential oil

Tools:

One 2 oz (60 ml) glass or PET plastic jar with a lid

Glass stirring rod

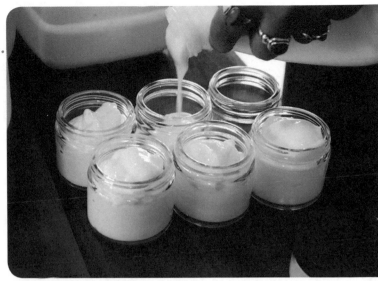

Pouring handmade lotion into jars at Aromahead Institute.

Moisturizing Facial Spray in Hydrosol *

Makes: One 1 oz (30 ml) spray bottle

Ingredients:

1 oz (30 ml) Rose hydrosol

1 drop Rose otto essential oil

2 drops Lavender essential oil

Tools:

One 1 oz (30 ml) plastic or glass spray bottle

Directions: Fill spray bottle with Rose hydrosol.

Add essential oil drops and shake to combine.

Notes: Use as a moisturizing toner after cleansing your face.

Directions: Fill empty jar with unscented lotion.

Add drops directly to lotion and stir for at least one minute.

Notes: It is always a good idea to test a facial blend on the inside of your wrist for a few hours to check for skin sensitivities. Apply to freshly cleaned skin at morning and night.

Oily Skin Moisturizer *

Makes: One 2 oz (60 ml) jar of moisturizer for the face

Ingredients:

2 oz (56 gm) organic unscented lotion

6 drops Rose otto essential oil

4 drops Frankincense essential oil

Tools:

One 2 oz (60 ml) glass or PET plastic jar with a lid

Glass stirring rod

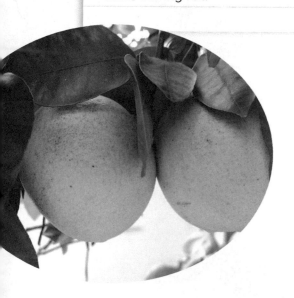

Directions: Fill empty jar with unscented lotion.

Add drops directly to lotion and stir for at least one minute.

Notes: It is always a good idea to test a facial blend on the inside of your wrist for a few hours to check for skin sensitivities. Apply to freshly cleansed skin at morning and night. Feel free to add one or two more drops of either oil if you prefer a stronger aroma.

Rosemary Shampoo Boost *

Makes: An uplifting, nourishing hair treatment

Ingredients:

Your favorite shampoo

Rosemary ct. verbenone essential oil

Directions: Squeeze your desired amount of shampoo into your palm.

Add one or two drops of Rosemary essential oil to the dollop of shampoo and wash as you normally would.

Rinse well before conditioning.

Notes: If you accidentally pour more than two drops, rinse your hand and start over. In large doses, Rosemary is too overpowering on your scalp. Avoid getting the shampoo and Rosemary essential oil into your eyes. We recommend using the Rosemary Shampoo Boost once a week.

Citrus Perfume Balm ***

Makes: Four 1 oz (30 ml) tins of hard perfume balm

Ingredients:

1 oz (28 gm) beeswax

3 oz (90 ml) jojoba oil

5 drops Orange essential oil

4 drops Petitgrain (Bigarade) essential oil

6 drops Neroli essential oil

Tools:

Kitchen scale

Large Pyrex measuring bowl

Medium stovetop pot

Glass stirring rod

Four 1 oz (30 ml) tins with lids

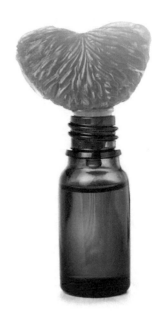

Directions: Use the Stovetop Melting Method to liquefy and combine the beeswax and jojoba oil.

After removing the jojoba and beeswax from the heat, add the essential oils and stir.

Pour into tins, add lids and allow to fully cool and harden before using. This should take at least an hour.

Notes: Soften with fingertip and apply balm to wrist and neck pulse points for a gentle, natural perfume.

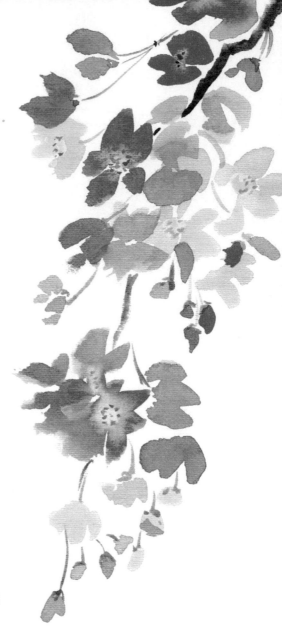

Floral Perfume Balm ***

Makes: Four 1 oz (30 ml) tins of hard perfume balm

Ingredients:

1 oz (28 gm) beeswax

3 oz (90 ml) jojoba oil

5 drops Rose absolute

2 drops Jasmine absolute

1 drop Palmarosa essential oil

Tools:

Kitchen scale

Large Pyrex measuring bowl

Medium stovetop pot

Glass stirring rod

Four 1 oz (30 ml) tins with lids

Directions: Use the Stovetop Melting Method to liquefy and combine the beeswax and jojoba oil.

After removing the jojoba and beeswax from the heat, add the essential oils and stir.

Pour into tins, add lids and allow to fully cool and harden before using. This should take at least an hour.

Notes: Soften with fingertip and apply balm to wrist and neck pulse points for a gentle, natural perfume.

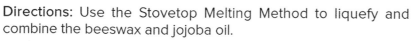

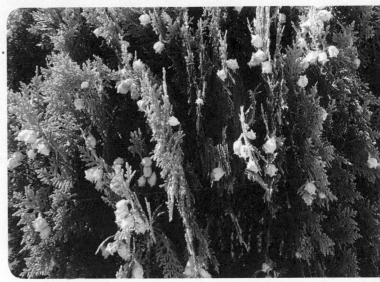

Cypress in Bulgaria.

Woodsy Perfume Balm ***

Makes: Four 1 oz (30 ml) tins of hard perfume balm

Ingredients:

1 oz (28 gm) beeswax

3 oz (90 ml) jojoba oil

5 drops Cypress essential oil

6 drops Juniper essential oil

6 drops Patchouli essential oil

Tools:

Kitchen scale

Large Pyrex measuring bowl

Medium stovetop pot

Glass stirring rod

Four 1 oz (30 ml) tins with lids

Directions: Use the Stovetop Melting Method to liquefy and combine the beeswax and jojoba oil.

After removing the jojoba and beeswax from the heat, add the essential oils and stir.

Pour into tins, add lids and allow to fully cool and harden before using. This should take at least an hour.

Notes: Soften with fingertip and apply balm to wrist and neck pulse points for a gentle, natural perfume.

Chapter 7 Medicine Chest

Your Aromatherapy Medicine Chest

What is the first thing you do when you have a cold? Do you head to the pharmacy to pick up a cold medication? Our society focuses strongly on treating and eliminating symptoms of various ailments and pains. Unfortunately, that can lead us to ignore the inherent causes of our problems.

Natural Healing and Prevention

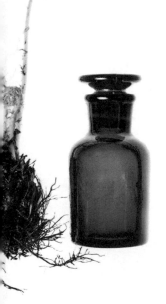

The first step toward using natural treatments is to become more in tune with your body and your symptoms. For example: Do you have a headache because you're stressed, because of allergies, or because of muscle soreness? With mindfulness and the assistance of a holistic or natural health care practitioner, you can begin to "wean" yourself and your children off of over-the-counter medications.

Many individuals can't replace every medication with a natural alternative, but many natural remedies can assist you with overall health. There are many simple, effective and natural preventative measures against common ailments like cold and flu.

These natural products are easy to use and make wonderful gifts for your loved ones. For instance, during cold and flu season, consider putting together a gift basket for your child's teacher or your coworkers.

Therapeutic Bath Salt for Aches and Pains *

Makes: One 8 oz (240 ml) jar of bath salts (enough for about 8 baths)

Ingredients:

8 oz (224 gm) natural (unbleached) bath salts

20 drops Saro essential oil

10 drops Patchouli essential oil

10 drops Frankincense essential oil

Tools:

One 8 oz (240 ml) PET plastic jar

Stirring spoon

Directions: Fill empty jar with bath salts.

Add essential oils directly to the salt and mix vigorously for at least one minute.

Notes: Add about 1 oz (28 gm) to your bath after the tub has filled. Soak and enjoy. Use to soothe the body after a vigorous workout or to relax and unwind after a tense day at work. We prefer pink Himalayan salt for use in the bath. Everyone loves the color.

Therapeutic Bath Salt for Cold and Flu *

Makes: One 8 oz (240 ml) jar of bath salts

(enough for about 8 baths)

Ingredients:

8 oz (224 gm) natural (unbleached) bath salts

20 drops Ravintsara essential oil

10 drops Gingergrass essential oil

10 drops Orange essential oil

Tools:

One 8 oz (240 ml) PET plastic jar

Stirring spoon

Directions: Fill empty jar with bath salts.

Add essential oils directly to the salt and mix vigorously for at least one minute.

Notes: Add about 1 oz (28 gm) to your bath after the tub has filled. Soak and enjoy. Use to relieve the aches, pains and discomfort associated with cold, cough and flu.

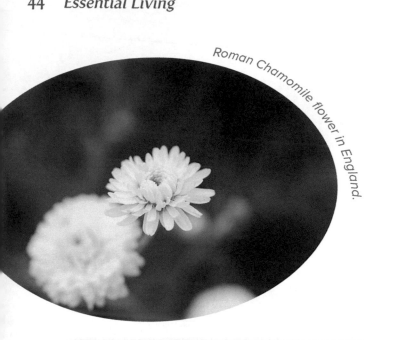

Roman Chamomile flower in England.

Directions: Fill empty jar with bath salts.

Add essential oils directly to the salt and mix vigorously for at least one minute.

Notes: Add about 1 oz (28 gm) to your bath after the tub has filled. Soak and enjoy. This blend is great to use just before bed.

Cooling Massage Oil for Pain Relief *

Makes: One 1 oz (30 ml) bottle of massage oil

Ingredients:

1 oz (30 ml) Trauma Oil (Trauma Oil contains Arnica, Calendula, and St. John's Wort.)

6 drops Gingergrass essential oil

6 drops Mandarin essential oil

8 drops Sandalwood essential oil

Tools:

One 1 oz (30 ml) PET plastic or glass bottle

Directions: Fill the empty bottle with 1 oz (30 ml) Trauma Oil.

Add the essential oils, screw cap tightly and shake to stir.

Notes: Use during massage for hot aches and pains. Great for acute muscle pain and injury and to reduce swelling.

Therapeutic Bath Salt for Sleep and Calm *

Makes: One 8 oz (240 ml) jar of bath salts

(enough for about 8 baths)

Ingredients:

8 oz (224 gm) natural (unbleached) bath salts

20 drops Roman Chamomile essential oil

20 drops Lavender essential oil

Tools:

One 8 oz (240 ml) PET plastic jar

Stirring spoon

Warming Massage Oil for Pain Relief *

Makes: One 1 oz (30 ml) bottle of massage oil

Ingredients:

1 oz (30 ml) Trauma Oil

6 drops Ginger essential oil

8 drops Myrrh essential oil

6 drops Elemi essential oil

Tools:

One 1 oz (30 ml) PET plastic or glass bottle

Directions: Fill the empty bottle with 1 oz (30 ml) Trauma Oil.

Add the essential oils, screw cap tightly and shake to stir.

Notes: Use during massage for tight, tense muscle aches. This warming oil works best on areas of the body experiencing stiff, stagnant pain. Great for arthritis.

Cleansing Diffuser Blend *

Makes: One 5 ml stock blend for use in a diffuser

Ingredients:

15 drops Norway Pine essential oil

15 drops Lemon essential oil

20 drops Lavender essential oil

Tools:

One 5 ml glass bottle with orifice reducer cap

Essential oil diffuser

Directions: Fill the small glass bottle with the three essential oils.

Label and store this stock blend in a cool, dark place.

Add 10 drops to your diffuser.

Notes: This blend is wonderful to diffuse when someone in your home is sick. It offers therapeutic relief while helping prevent the spread of airborne germs.

This blend is appropriate for day or night use.

Eczema and Dry Skin Balm ***

Makes: Four to five 1 oz (30 ml) glass jars of healing balm (depending on how high you fill them)

Ingredients:

1 oz (30 ml) avocado oil

1 oz (30 ml) jojoba oil

1.5 oz (45 ml) rose hip seed oil

1 oz (28 gm) beeswax

.25 teaspoon liquid Vitamin E

Tools:

Kitchen scale

Large Pyrex measuring bowl

Medium stovetop pot

Glass stirring rod

Four 1 oz (30 ml) jars with screw-on lids

Directions: Use the Stovetop Melting Method to liquefy and combine the beeswax and jojoba oils.

Remove the combined oils from the heat and add the remaining ingredients.

Stir and pour into the jars.

Add lids and allow to fully cool and harden before using. This should take at least an hour.

Notes: Apply liberally to dry skin directly after bath while skin is still slightly damp.

Headache Relief Oil *

Makes: One 1 oz (30 ml) jar of headache relief oil

Ingredients:

1 oz (30 ml) jojoba oil

7 drops Peppermint essential oil

5 drops Frankincense essential oil

3 drops Lemon essential oil

Tools:

One 1 oz (30 ml) glass or PET plastic jar with screw top

Directions: Fill empty jar with 1 oz (30 ml) jojoba.

Add oils directly to jar.

Screw lid on carefully, shake to mix.

Notes: Shake before use. Apply to the back of neck or shoulders at onset of headache. Avoid using directly on the face and keep away from eyes. Always wash hands after applying.

Apply every 15 minutes for an hour.

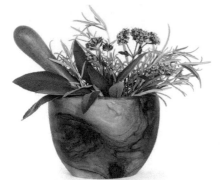

Nasal Congestion Relief Inhaler *

Makes: One therapeutic Aromatherapy inhaler

Ingredients:

5 drops Eucalyptus globulus

5 drops White Pine

5 drops Ravintsara

Tools:

One blank Aromatherapy inhaler

Directions: Add drops directly to the blank cotton component of the Aromatherapy inhaler.

Attach lid carefully.

Notes: Use as needed to relieve congestion and pain associated with sinus colds. To avoid the spread of germs, Aromatherapy inhalers should be used by one person only.

Steam Blend for Sinus Relief *

Makes: One 5 ml stock blend for sinus steams

Ingredients:

20 drops Eucalyptus dives essential oil

20 drops Saro essential oil

10 drops White Pine essential oil

Tools:

One 5 ml glass bottle with orifice reducer cap

Directions: Fill the small glass bottle with the three essential oils.

Label and store this stock blend in a cool, dark place.

Use as needed for steam treatments or in a diffuser.

Notes: This blend is used to relieve the pain, congestion and swelling associated with sinus colds and sinus headaches.

Always use one drop and keep your eyes closed when using neat essential oil blends in a steam treatment. For added benefit, leave the bowl of steaming water out—the oils will continue to diffuse.

If you experience discomfort or nasal irritation, avoid use in steam and diffuse instead.

Chapter 8 The Living Room

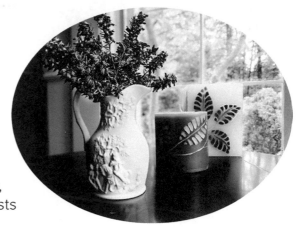

A Naturally Inviting Living Room

Have you ever walked into a home that simply felt cozy to you? It may have been because of the decorations in the house, or the aroma of cookies in the oven, or a satchel of potpourri that reminded you of your grandmother's house. Natural Aromatherapy helps you create a cozy, inviting atmosphere in your home for your guests and your family.

Aroma and Atmosphere

The diffuser blends you create can be used throughout the year, depending on your mood or the atmosphere you'd like to set in your home. Feel free to adjust them as you become more familiar with essential oils and as your collection expands.

Note: If you're using a candle diffuser be sure to add warm water to the bowl along with your essential oil diffuser blend.

The cleaning products in this chapter are gentle, chemical-free alternatives to common household cleaning products. As with the bathroom products, they're effective and safe, with ingredients you'll recognize without needing a chemistry degree.

The potpourri sachet makes a perfect gift or stocking stuffer. Consider creating them as housewarming gifts, bridal shower gifts, or as a simple thank you for a friend. As with the diffuser blends, potpourri can be adjusted and customized as you become more comfortable blending essential oils.

Calming Diffuser Blend *

Makes: One 5 ml stock blend for use in a diffuser

Ingredients:

20 drops Ho Wood essential oil

10 drops Petitgrain (Bigarade) essential oil

20 drops Lavender essential oil

Tools:

One 5 ml glass bottle with orifice

Reducer cap

Essential oil diffuser

Directions: Fill the small glass bottle with the three essential oils.

Label and store this stock blend in a cool, dark place.

Add 10 drops to your diffuser.

Notes: Use this blend to create a relaxing and calming atmosphere in your home. Great for times of stress or to calm little ones down before bedtime.

Energizing Diffuser Blend *

Makes: One 5 ml stock blend for use in a diffuser

Ingredients:

15 drops Rosemary ct. camphor essential oil

15 drops distilled Lime essential oil

15 drops Grapefruit essential oil

Tools:

One 5 ml glass bottle with orifice reducer cap

Essential oil diffuser

Directions: Fill the small glass bottle with the three essential oils.

Label and store this stock blend in a cool, dark place.

Add 10 drops to your diffuser.

Notes: Use this blend to create an uplifting and energizing atmosphere in your home. Because this blend is stimulating, It's best for use during the day. We love using this in the wintertime to brighten the day.

Wintertime Steam Diffuser Blend *

Makes: Warm, steamy aromatic mist

Ingredients:

5 drops Black Spruce essential oil

5 drops Balsam Fir essential oil

5 drops Grapefruit essential oil

Tools:

A small soup pan or teapot for use on a stove. You can also use this blend in a candle or electric diffuser.

Directions: Heat water to a low simmer. Then turn off the heat.

Add the oils and allow them to diffuse with the steam from the heated water.

Notes: This blend is specifically formulated for wintertime. The bright grapefruit aroma is light and emotionally uplifting. The conifer oils are wonderful for respiratory issues and can help combat winter colds and the flu.

Rose petals drying in Bulgaria.

Hydrosol Upholstery Spray *

Makes: One bottle of aromatic spray for upholstery freshening

Ingredients:

Organic Lavender hydrosol

Tools:

If your hydrosol did not come with a spray lid, transfer it to a clean spray bottle.

Directions: Mist upholstery lightly to freshen and to add a subtle scent of calming lavender.

Notes: Only spray this on materials that can tolerate small amounts of water or a damp cloth. Use this to freshen up during regular cleanings or after guests have been in the home.

Potpourri Sachet *

Makes: One sachet of aromatic potpourri

Ingredients:

1/2 cup dried herbs (such as dried lavender, dried rose petals)

4 drops Rose otto essential oil

15 drops Orange essential oil

Tools (Optional):

Small mesh or cloth bag with tie opening

Directions: Add drops of essential oils to dry herbs.

Stir and mix to spread oil around evenly.

Notes: This potpourri blend can be used in a small bowl to diffuse the scent in a small room. Alternatively, try using a small mesh or cloth bag with a decorative tie. This makes a lovely bathroom scent.

Window Cleaner *

Makes: One 16 oz (480 ml) spray bottle of window cleaner with a gentle lavender aroma

Ingredients:

14 oz (420 ml) water

2 tablespoons white vinegar

2 tablespoon Lavender hydrosol

50 drops Lavender essential oil

Tools:

One 16 oz (480 ml) spray bottle

Directions: Mix all ingredients in spray bottle. Add oils last.

Notes: Shake liberally before using. Clean windows with paper towels, cloth or newspaper. This spray can be used on any hard surface, and makes a wonderful all purpose spray for kitchens and bathrooms.

Wood Polish ***

Makes: One 4 oz (120 ml) bottle of hard polish for wood floors

Ingredients:

1 oz (28 gm) beeswax

3 oz (90 ml) jojoba oil

30 drops Siberian Fir essential oil

Tools:

Kitchen scale

Pyrex style large measuring bowl

Medium stovetop pot

Glass stirring rod

One 4 oz (120 ml) glass jar with lid

Directions: Use the Stovetop Melting Method to liquefy and combine the beeswax and jojoba oil.

After removing from the heat, add the essential oils and stir.

Pour into jar, add lid and allow to fully cool and harden before using. This should take at least an hour.

Notes: Use a clean cloth or rag to spread a small amount of the polish vigorously over wood. Use a second clean cloth to remove all excess polish. There should be no excess greasiness.

Chapter 9 The Bedroom

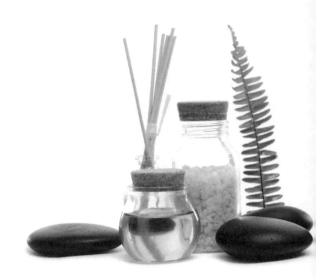

Aromatherapy Relief in the Bedroom

Researchers have attributed a host of health concerns to lack of sleep. Problems ranging from poor job performance to frequent illnesses may stem from not getting enough good sleep at night. Those who struggle with sleep issues are often desperate for ways to get a better night's sleep.

Peaceful Sleep and Relaxation

Natural Aromatherapy recipes for the bedroom include blends to assist with calming down, falling asleep and staying asleep. We've also included blends to help you sleep when you have cold and flu symptoms.

Make your bedtime a ritual and incorporate your favorite Aromatherapy blends into this ritual. You might follow up a soothing bath with an application of a calming body spray or with jojoba oil mixed with a sleep blend. Or you might take time to turn down your sheets and spritz them with a hydrosol linen spray.

Aromatherapy alone won't always give you a great night's sleep. Remember to avoid having a television on or bright lights on in your room. Create an atmosphere that appeals to you, whether that means white noise, music, or silence. Give yourself enough time to fall asleep, and avoid caffeine and stimulating essential oils in the evening before bedtime.

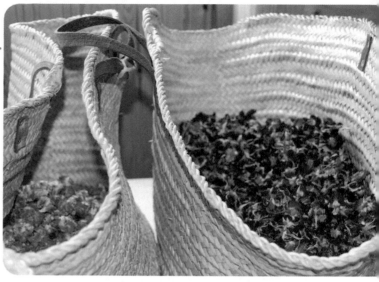

Dried roses in France.

Calming Body Spray *

Makes: One 4 oz (120 ml) bottle of calming body spray

Ingredients:

5 drops Lemongrass essential oil

16 drops Gingergrass essential oil

2 drops Rose otto essential oil

4 oz (120 ml) water

Tools:

One 4 oz (120 ml) spray bottle

Directions: Add oils to water in spray bottle, shake gentle to mix.

Notes: Shake gently before use. Avoid spraying directly to the face. Try spraying onto your clothes or torso for a gently calming affect. This spray can also be soothing in hot weather.

Hydrosol Linen Spray *

Makes: One bottle of aromatic linen spray

Ingredients:

Organic Sweetgrass hydrosol

Tools:

If your hydrosol did not come with a spray lid, transfer it to a clean spray bottle.

Directions: Mist linens lightly to freshen and add the subtle scent of freshly cut grass.

Notes: Try using this linen spray before bedtime, when traveling in hotels, or to refresh linens that have been in storage.

Nighttime Cold Relief Blend in Jojoba *

Makes: One 1 oz (30 ml) bottle of soothing oil for skin

Ingredients:

1 oz (30 ml) jojoba oil

5 drops Lavender essential oil

5 drops Lemon essential oil

3 drops Roman Chamomile essential oil

Tools:

One 1 oz (30 ml) glass or PET plastic bottle

Directions: Add oils to jojoba in bottle, shake gently to mix.

Notes: Shake gently before use. Apply to the back of the neck, chest and feet as needed in evenings and at bedtime. Try keeping this blend on the nightstand.

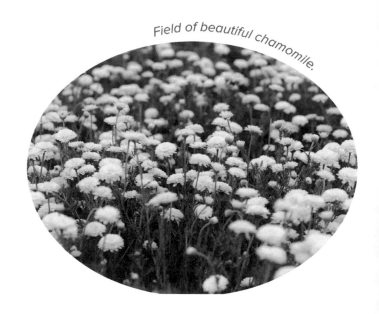

Field of beautiful chamomile.

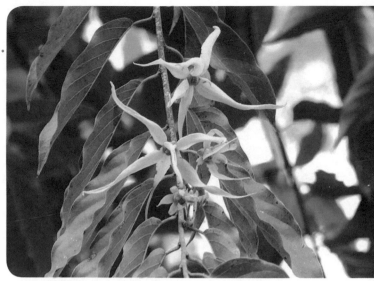

Ylang Ylang flowers from our tree in Florida, USA.

Exotic Diffuser Blend *

Makes: An inviting atmosphere using essential oils in a diffuser

Ingredients:

2 drops Ylang Ylang essential oil

1 drop Neroli essential oil

3 drops Patchouli essential oil

Tools:

Essential oil diffuser

Directions: Add the oils to your favorite diffuser and enjoy.

Notes: If you do not have neroli on hand, try using jasmine. If you don't enjoy the aroma of patchouli, try substituting with your favorite base note such as a spikenard or vetiver.

Sleep Blend in Jojoba Oil *

Makes: One 1 oz (30 ml) bottle of calming sleep oil for skin

Ingredients:

1 oz (30 ml) jojoba oil

5 drops Ylang Ylang essential oil

5 drops Lavender essential oil

Tools:

One 1 oz (30 ml) glass or PET plastic bottle.

Directions: Add oils to jojoba in the 1 oz (30 ml) bottle. Shake gently to combine.

Notes: Apply to the back of neck and feet ten minutes before bedtime.

Chapter 10 Caring for Kids

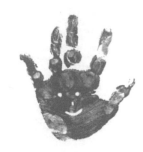

Limiting Exposure to Toxins and Chemicals

Babies and children are far more susceptible to environmental toxins than adults are. They eat more food per pound than adults, they tend to put their hands and toys in their mouths and they're growing and developing at a rapid rate compared to adults. As parents and caretakers, we can create a healthier environment for kids by limiting exposure to toxins and synthetic chemicals.

Gentle Remedies, Safe Cleaning

The use of Aromatherapy, hand-made cleaning products and natural remedies can help limit the use of chemicals in the home. The next step is to create products made **specifically for use with children**. The blends in this chapter give you natural alternatives to everyday products like antibacterial hand gel, moisturizing balm and diaper pail spray.

These blends have been specially formulated for the safety standards used when blending for young children. The bathroom relaxation blend in jojoba is a natural, safe alternative to "nighttime" bubble bath brands that actually contain a synthetic version of lavender that's harmful to children with sensitive skin and that may contain concerning chemicals.

We've also included a diffuser blend to help kids calm down and focus. This is perfect for preschool-aged children who have a tendency to get wound up before bedtime, and for older kids who need a little boost at homework time. These natural alternatives have been a tremendous help for some parents with children who struggle with attention span issues and hyperactivity.

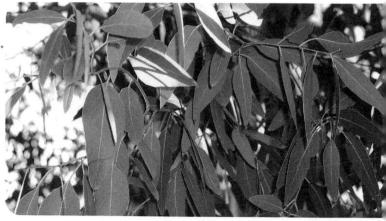

Eucalyptus leaves in Greece.

Antibacterial Diffuser Blend *

Makes: One 5 ml stock blend for use in a diffuser

Ingredients:

20 drops Cedarwood essential oil

20 drops Orange essential oil

20 drops Balsam Fir essential oil

Tools:

One 5 ml glass bottle with orifice

Reducer cap

Essential oil diffuser

Directions: Fill the small glass bottle with the three essential oils.

Label and store this stock blend in a cool, dark place.

Add 10 drops to your diffuser.

Notes: Diffuse this blend when you or your children are experiencing cold or flu symptoms. This blend is wonderful to diffuse in the living room or other highly trafficked areas. It can also be used to clear the air after guests have been in the home or after a play date.

Gentle Back Rub Oil for Cough and Colds*

Makes: One 1 oz (30 ml) bottle of oil to combat the symptoms of cold and cough

Ingredients:

1 oz (30 ml) jojoba oil

3 drops Roman Chamomile essential oil

3 drops Balsam Fir essential oil

Tools:

One 1 oz (30 ml) glass or PET plastic bottle

Directions: Add oils to jojoba in bottle, shake gently to mix.

Notes: Shake gently before use. Apply to the back of the neck and back before bedtime or as needed during the day. Try applying this blend in a steamy bathroom to help carry the soothing vapors.

Not for use on children under five.

Bathtime Relaxation Blend in Jojoba *

Makes: One 4 oz (120 ml) PET plastic bottle of oil for the bath

Ingredients:

4 oz (120 ml) jojoba oil

20 drops Spikenard essential oil

10 drops Orange essential oil

Tools:

One 4 oz (120 ml) PET plastic bottle

Directions: Add oils to jojoba in bottle, shake gently to mix.

Notes: Add a small capful of this bath oil to running bathwater. The jojoba oil gently moisturizes while the spikenard and orange work together to calm and soothe the nerves. Wipe the tub with a clean towel after draining to avoid slippery residue from the jojoba oil.

Not for use on children under five.

Calm and Focus Diffuser Blend *

Makes: One 5 ml stock blend for use in a diffuser

Ingredients:

25 drops Orange essential oil

25 drops Lavender essential oil

Tools:

One 5 ml glass bottle with orifice reducer cap

Essential oil diffuser

Directions: Fill the small glass bottle with the two essential oils.

Label and store this stock blend in a cool, dark place.

Add 10 drops to your diffuser.

Notes: Diffuse this blend as your child is working on homework or tasks that require focus. This blend can be great to use to create a calming atmosphere after a hectic or stimulating day.

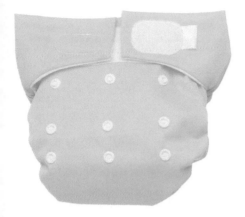

Diaper Pail Spray *

Makes: One 4 oz (120 ml) spray bottle of deodorizing & cleansing spray for the diaper changing area

Ingredients:

4 oz (120 ml) water

15 drops White Pine essential oil

15 drops Lemon essential oil

Tools:

One 4 oz (120 ml) PET plastic spray bottle

Directions: Add oils to the water in bottle, shake gently to mix.

Notes: Shake before using. Spray liberally onto the diaper pail and onto any plastic surfaces around the diaper changing area. This spray is not for use on the skin. Avoid spraying directly onto the changing pad as baby's bare skin may come in contact with it.

Cloth Diaper Laundry Booster *

Makes: Natural essential oil laundry boosters for use in cloth diaper laundering

Ingredients:

4 drops Tea Tree essential oil

4 drops Lavender essential oil

Directions:

Add the tea tree and lavender oil to the soaking cycle of your washing machine.

Notes: Tea tree oil helps to disinfect dirty diapers as they soak. Lavender gives the diapers a subtle, fresh aroma as they rinse.

Cleansing Hand Gel for Caretakers and Kids **

Makes: One 4 oz (120 ml) spray bottle of natural, chemical-free, cleansing hand gel

Ingredients:

4 oz (112 gm) organic aloe vera gel

4 drops Tea Tree essential oil

8 drops Cedarwood essential oil

8 drops Orange essential oil

Tools:

One 4 oz (120 ml) PET plastic spray bottle

Directions: Add oils to the aloe vera gel, shake vigorously to combine.

Notes: Apply liberally to hands and rub until the gel has evaporated. This can be stored in the fridge and transferred into convenient 1 oz (30 ml) spray bottles to keep in your purse or diaper bag for hand cleansing on the go. Store extra gel in the fridge if you make a large amount ahead of time.

Avoid purchasing aloe with extra ingredients. A small amount of natural preservative is fine.

Not for children under five.

Hydrosol Skin Calming Spray *

Makes: One 4 oz (120 ml) spray for the skin

Ingredients:

4 oz (120 ml) organic Sweetgrass hydrosol

2 drops Lavender essential oil

Tools:

One 4 oz (120 ml) spray bottle

Directions: Mix the drops of essential oil with the hydrosol. Shake gently to combine.

Notes: Shake before use. Mist dry or irritated skin lightly. Do not use on face. This spray is great to use after exposure to the sun or cold winter air.

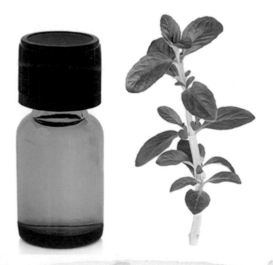

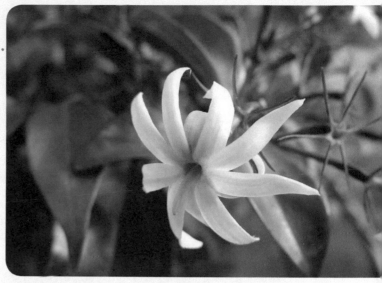

Fragrant jasmine flower in Florida.

Little Lips and Cheek Balm **

Makes: Four 1 oz (30 ml) tins of soothing balm

Ingredients:

1 oz (28 gm) beeswax

3 oz (84 gm) coconut oil

Tools:

Kitchen scale

Large Pyrex measuring bowl

Medium stovetop pot

Glass stirring rod

Four 1 oz (30 ml) tins with screw-on lids

Directions: Use the Stovetop Melting Method to liquefy and combine the beeswax and coconut oils.

Remove the combined beeswax and coconut oil from heat and pour into the tins.

Add lids and allow to fully cool and harden before using. This should take at least an hour.

Notes: Apply to cheeks and lips to soothe dry skin, protect skin from wind and cold weather, and calm skin after exposure to the sun. Note: This balm can be used in the diaper area, but if you choose to do so, be sure to avoid contaminating the balm.

Chapter II   The Office

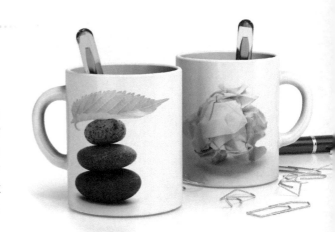

Take Your Essential Oils to Work

Whether your office is a cubicle, a kitchen table or the driver's seat, chances are you encounter some work stress. Many of us carry work home every day, literally and emotionally. We also carry germs home. Our recipes for the office are perfect for fighting the pain, stress and illness that can stem from the workplace.

Before you work on these blends, take time to consider your personal work situation. What aspects of it are satisfying to you? Which aspects are stressful? Do you find yourself frequently taking pain relievers or frequently becoming ill? After you step back and evaluate your relationship with your career, you'll have a better understanding of how natural blends might benefit you.

Pain Relief, Stress Management

The cleansing hand moisturizer can be your best tool against the spread of germs in the office. Keep it on your desk next to your keyboard. Remember to use it to clean your hands after you've used someone else's computer or equipment. If you work on the go, keep it with you in your purse or even in the car.

Aromatherapy inhalers are convenient ways to enjoy Aromatherapy in atmospheres where you can't diffuse essential oils. Keep the inhaler in your pocket for quick access to stress relieving or immune boosting blends.

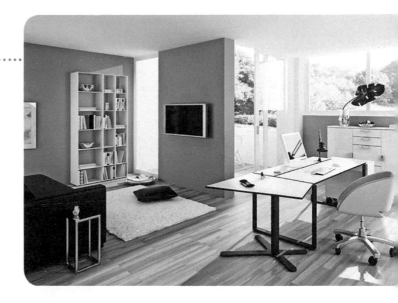

If you work at the computer or you find yourself frequently stressed, the tension headache relief blend can work wonders. The aroma is subtle enough that it shouldn't affect or bother your coworkers—which is more than we can say for most synthetic perfumes and colognes!

Cleansing Hand Moisturizer *

Makes: 2 oz (60 ml) PET plastic spray bottle of hand moisturizer

Ingredients:

2 oz (56 gm) organic aloe vera gel

20 drops Lavender essential oil

Tools:

2 oz (60 ml) PET plastic spray bottle

Directions: Add the aloe vera to the spray bottle then add the drops of lavender essential oil.

Shake to mix.

Notes: Spray each hand three or four times. Rub briskly until the liquid dries.

Keep near your keyboard and use frequently to fight office germs.

Immune Boosting Inhaler *

Makes: One therapeutic Aromatherapy inhaler

Ingredients:

5 drops Ravintsara essential oil

5 drops Tea Tree essential oil

5 drops Eucalyptus radiata essential oil

Tools:

One blank Aromatherapy inhaler

Directions: Add drops directly to the blank cotton component of the Aromatherapy inhaler.

Attach lid carefully.

Notes: Breathe into each nostril several times a day for a healthy immune-boosting dose of essential oils. Try keeping one in the office and another in the car.

Stress Relief Inhaler *

Makes: One therapeutic Aromatherapy inhaler

Ingredients:

8 drops Bergamot Mint essential Oil

8 drops Orange essential oil

Tools:

One blank Aromatherapy inhaler

Directions: Add drops directly to the blank cotton component of the Aromatherapy inhaler.

Attach lid carefully.

Notes: Breathe into each nostril as needed. This can be particularly effective at times of stress and anxiety. Use it for a moment of peace and serenity before a big presentation or after a tense meeting.

Soothing Lip Balm ***

Makes: Four 1 oz (30 ml) tins of lip balm

Ingredients:

1 oz (28 gm) beeswax

3 oz (84 gm) coconut oil

32 drops of Orange essential oil

Tools:

Kitchen scale

Large Pyrex measuring bowl

Medium stovetop pot

Glass stirring rod

Four 1 oz (30 ml) tins with screw-on lids

Directions: Use the Stovetop Melting Method to liquefy and combine the beeswax and coconut oils.

Add the 32 drops of orange essential oil and quickly mix.

Remove the combined oils and beeswax from heat and pour into the tins.

Add lids and allow to fully cool and harden before using. This should take at least an hour.

Notes: Apply to lips several times a day to combat the effects of dry air and air conditioning in the office. Orange essential oil soothes the skin and provides a gentle antibacterial effect.

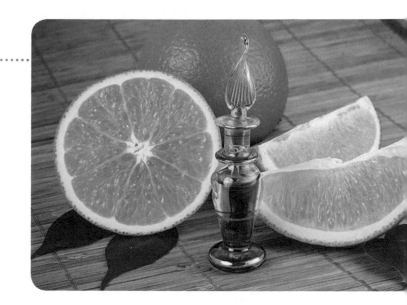

Tension Headache Relief Oil *

Makes: One 1 oz (30 ml) bottle of tension headache relief oil

Ingredients:

1 oz (30 ml) jojoba oil

5 drops Peppermint essential oil

10 drops Orange essential oil

Tools:

One 1 oz (30 ml) glass or PET plastic bottle with a flip top

Directions: Fill empty bottle with 1 oz (30 ml) jojoba.

Add oils directly to jar.

Screw lid on carefully, shake to mix.

Notes: Shake before use. Apply to the back of neck or shoulders at onset of headache. Avoid using directly on the face and keep away from eyes. Always wash hands after applying.

Apply every 15 minutes for an hour.

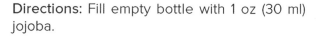

Chapter 12 Patios & Outdoor Spaces

Enjoy the Outdoors

Depending on where you live, bugs may be a seasonal issue or may be something you deal with year round. We use essential oils in all of our cleaning and pest management. The recipes in our patio section help you clean and maintain your outdoor spaces.

Eucalyptus leaves.

Outdoors pests and insects don't need to be killed with harsh chemicals. Our pest blends for use outdoors help combat insects without exposing your plants, animals or children to toxic chemicals. It's important to remember that we share outdoor spaces with natural wildlife and bugs. We can't eradicate every bug or potential annoyance, but we can help make spaces more people-friendly.

Bug Control, Seasonal Cleaning

Keep in mind that natural bug repellents need to be used more liberally and applied more often than bug sprays that contain chemicals. Also think about wearing long sleeves, long pants and socks. This will help you minimize exposed skin for bugs to chew on!

When it comes to cleaning outside, always be prepared to use a little extra elbow grease. Mildew and other seasonal discolorations require serious scrubbing. Use a heavy, abrasive rag or scrubbing pad with our outdoor furniture cleaning spray.

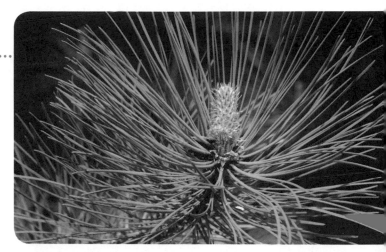

Pine needles.

Natural Bug Repellent *

Makes: One 4 oz (120 ml) bottle of repellent spray

Ingredients:

4 oz (120 ml) water

20 drops Cedarwood essential oil

15 drops Eucalyptus citriodora essential oil

10 drops Patchouli essential oil

5 drops Lavender essential oil

Tools:

One 4 oz (120 ml) PET plastic spray bottle

Directions: Add the water to the spray bottle.

Add the essential oils.

Shake well to mix.

Notes: Shake before using. Because this bug spray does not contain pesticides, it needs to be re-applied frequently. Spray skin and clothes every hour. Do not spray the face directly. You can spray your hands and wipe them onto your face, but avoid using on the hands and faces of young children and babies.

Outdoor Furniture Scrub Spray *

Makes: One 8 oz (240 ml) spray bottle

Ingredients:

7.5 oz (225 ml) water

2 tablespoons white vinegar

20 drops White Pine essential oil

20 drops Lemon essential oil

20 drops Juniper essential oil

Tools:

One 8 oz (240 ml) spray bottle

Directions: Pour the water and vinegar into the spray bottle.

Add the essential oils.

Shake well to mix.

Notes: Shake before using. Spray patio furniture liberally. Clean and scrub with a heavy rag. Avoid spraying directly onto the skin.

Itch Stick ***

Makes: Twelve 5 ml lip balm tubes of itch relief sticks

Ingredients:

.5 oz (15 ml) jojoba oil

1 oz (28 gm) coconut oil

.5 oz (14 gm) beeswax

15 drops Lavender essential oil

15 drops Helichrysum italicum essential oil

5 drops Peppermint essential oil

Tools:

Kitchen scale

Large Pyrex measuring bowl

Medium stovetop pot

Glass stirring rod

Twelve 5 ml lip balm tubes

Lip balm tube tray

Plastic pipettes

Directions: Use the Stovetop Melting Method to liquefy and combine the beeswax, jojoba and coconut oils.

Add the essential oils after the beeswax and carrier oils have combined.

Remove the combined oils and beeswax from the heat.

Immediately and carefully squirt the liquid balm into the lip balm tubes using plastic pipettes. If the liquid begins to solidify before you're finished transferring it to the tubes, simply place back onto heat.

Allow to fully cool and harden before using. This should take at least an hour.

Notes: Apply to raised welts, bumps and itchy bites as needed.

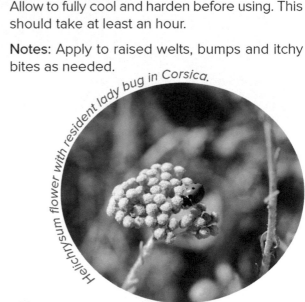

Helichrysum flower with resident lady bug in *Corsica.*

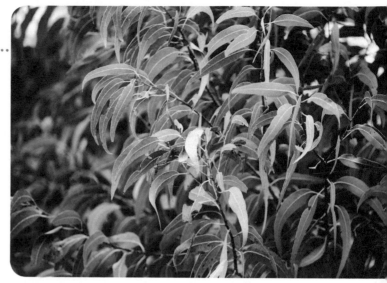

Eucalyptus leaves in Florida, USA.

Ant and Pest Spray *

Makes: One 4 oz (120 ml) spray bottle of household pest spray

Ingredients:

4 oz (120 ml) water

20 drops Peppermint essential oil

15 drops Eucalyptus citriodora essential oil

Tools:

One 4 oz (120 ml) PET plastic spray bottle

Directions: Add the water to the spray bottle.

Add the essential oils.

Shake well to mix.

Notes: Spray surfaces and nook and crannies liberally. Wipe with a clean towel until damp.

Use every day until pests have subsided.

Chapter 13 Travel

Boost Your Immune System on the Road

Travel exposes you to germs and stress you might not encounter at home. Enclosed spaces, disrupted sleep schedules and exposure to crowds can all make you more susceptible to illness and discomfort. Next time you prepare to travel, put a kit of essential oil blends together that will help boost your immune system, fight germs and keep your stress levels manageable.

Essential Travel Kit

Both inhalers in this chapter can be easily tucked into a pocket or purse for on-the-go relief. Use them to calm down during an airline flight, in traffic or even if you're feeling a little nervous meeting new people (or your in-laws). The immune system boosting inhaler is a must-have for time spent on public transportation. We find it's also wonderful for clearing the sinuses when you're exposed to allergens in an environment you're not used to.

The hand cleanser is great for when you're on the go. Use it when you're visiting tourist attractions and when you've been touching surfaces in crowded spaces like public transportation and shopping areas. The travel salve is your final secret weapon. Use it as a first defense against bruises, chapping, sunburn, sore muscles or even on the back of the neck as headache relief.

Try to make yourself at home when you travel. Use the linen spray on hotel sheets, try using music or ambient noise to help you sleep, and pay attention to all of your senses.

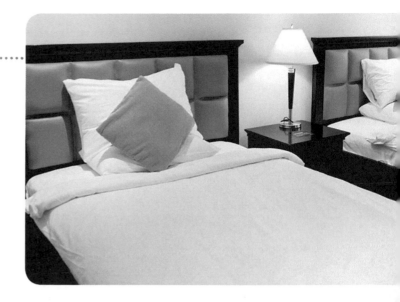

Some travelers find it beneficial to use a small worry stone or other object to keep fingers busy and soothed during times of stress while traveling. If you're a nervous traveler, don't be afraid to develop your own tricks, and remember to bring your inhaler!

Anxiety Relief Inhaler *

Makes: One therapeutic Aromatherapy inhaler

Ingredients:

10 drops Frankincense essential oil

5 drops Cypress essential oil

Tools:

One blank Aromatherapy inhaler

Directions: Add drops directly to the blank cotton component of the Aromatherapy inhaler.

Attach lid carefully.

Notes: Breathe into each nostril as needed. Keep in your pocket on airline flights. Breathe deeply, close your eyes, and focus on the grounding and calming aromas.

Crowded Spaces Immunity Inhaler *

Makes: One therapeutic Aromatherapy inhaler

Ingredients:

7 drops Ravintsara essential oil

8 drops White Pine essential oil

Tools:

One blank Aromatherapy inhaler

Directions: Add drops directly to the blank cotton component of the Aromatherapy inhaler.

Attach lid carefully.

Notes: Breathe into each nostril as needed. These immune boosting essential oils can help fight cold and flu germs in crowded spaces like airliners and public transportation.

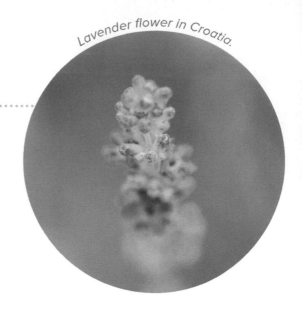

Lavender flower in Croatia.

Hand Cleansing Gel for Travel *

Makes: 2 oz (60 ml) PET plastic spray bottle of hand cleansing gel

Ingredients:

2 oz (56 gm) organic aloe vera gel

5 drops Peppermint essential oil

10 drops Lavender essential oil

5 drops Tea Tree essential oil

Tools:

2 oz (60 ml) PET plastic spray bottle

Directions: Add the aloe vera to the spray bottle then add the essential oils.

Shake to mix.

Notes: Spray each hand three or four times. Rub briskly until the liquid dries. Try using immediately after disembarking from flights or public transportation.

Hotel Linen Spray *

Makes: One 2 oz (60 ml) bottle of gently cleansing linen spray

Ingredients:

2 oz (60 ml) organic Lavender hydrosol

5 drops Tea Tree essential oil

5 drops Ravintsara essential oil

5 drops White Pine essential oil

Tools:

2 oz (60 ml) PET plastic spray bottle

Directions: Add essential oils to the hydrosol in the spray bottle. Shake to mix.

Notes: Shake before using. First, remove comforter from the hotel bed. Then mist the hotel sheets and pillow liberally, allowing time to dry before bed.

Travel Salve for Skin ***

Makes: Three 1 oz (30 ml) tins of hard salve

Ingredients:

2 oz (60 ml) Trauma Oil

1 oz (28 gm) beeswax

20 drops Peppermint essential oil

20 drops Lavender essential oil

Tools:

Kitchen scale

Large Pyrex measuring bowl

Medium stovetop pot

Glass stirring rod

Three 1 oz (30 ml) tins with lids

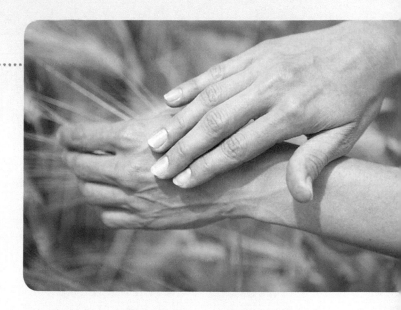

Directions: Use the Stovetop Melting Method to liquefy and combine the beeswax and Trauma Oil.

After removing from the heat, add the essential oils and stir.

Pour into tins, add lids and allow to fully cool and harden before using. This should take at least an hour.

Notes: This soothing, all-purpose salve can be used on many ailments while traveling. Use on bruises, for stiff muscles or for inflammation. This can also be used to help heal dry, cracked skin.

Chapter 14   Emotional Well Being

Focus and Overcome Stress

Every individual has a personal way of enhancing well being. For some, that might mean an exercise routine. For others, it might mean spending time gardening or going on quiet walks. We find joy where we can and cope with life's stressful moments in a variety of ways. Essential oils can assist with focusing the mind and facilitating healing. This chapter offers three very simple blends to incorporate into your personal routines.

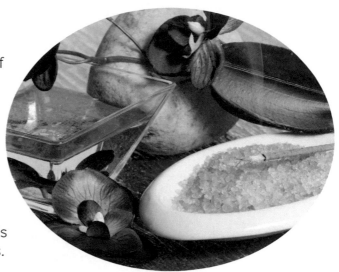

Supporting Mental Health

Don't feel limited to the three blends in this chapter. Essential oils can be used to support your emotional well being and mental health in many ways. Sometimes it's as simple as diffusing an aroma you love or wearing a blend with calming base notes when you meditate. Use these three blends as your foundation and build from there as you discover what your body and mind respond to.

When using essential oils for your mood, rely on a combination of basics and the way they make you feel. For example, citrus aromas are naturally bright, airy and uplifting while deep base notes from resins are calming, centering and grounding.

While we can identify through experience and science that certain essential oils have certain effects on your emotional state, it still comes down to individual experience and response. You may end up tweaking these blends or creating your own blends to help you focus, reduce negative feelings or to calm down in times of anxiety.

Focus & Concentration Inhaler *

Makes: One therapeutic Aromatherapy inhaler

Ingredients:

5 drops Rosemary ct camphor essential oil

10 drops Lemon essential oil

Tools:

One blank Aromatherapy inhaler

Directions: Add drops directly to the blank cotton component of the Aromatherapy inhaler.

Attach lid carefully.

Notes: Use while working or studying to assist with focus and concentration.

Stress Relief Body Spray *

Makes: One 4 oz (120 ml) bottle of stress relieving body spray

Ingredients:

4 oz (120 ml) water

6 drops Ylang Ylang essential oil

4 drops Neroli essential oil

Tools:

One 4 oz (120 ml) PET plastic or glass spray bottle

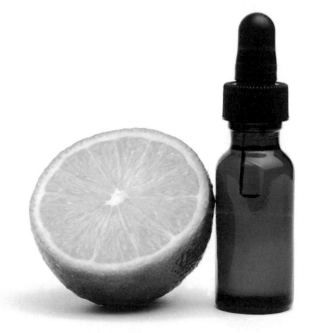

Directions: Add oils to water in spray bottle, shake gentle to mix.

Notes: Shake gently before use. Avoid spraying directly on the face. Try keeping it in the refrigerator and then using it as a soothing mist just before bed. Alternatively, it can be sprayed on the sheets and pillow before bed.

This body spray has a floral, feminine aroma.

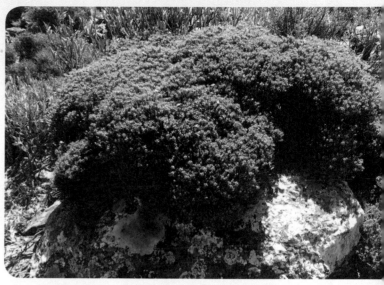

Thyme growing along the side of the road in Greece.

Antidepressant Room Spray *

Makes: One 2 oz (60 ml) bottle of therapeutic room spray

Ingredients:

2 oz (60 ml) water

5 drops Ylang Ylang essential oil

10 drops Orange essential oil

2 drops distilled Lime essential oil

Tools:

One 2 oz (60 ml) PET plastic spray bottle

Directions: Add oils to the water in bottle, shake gently to mix.

Notes: Shake before using. Spray into the air in the living room and bedroom. The gentle floral aroma and bright citrus oils offer a supportive, antidepressant effect.

Chapter 15   Aromatic indulgences

Your Relationship with Aromatherapy

As you become more familiar with your collection of essential oils, you will begin to see them as faithful friends. Lemon might be your partner on days when you feel down. Lavender might be your helper when you're wound up and need help getting to sleep. You may develop a special affinity for certain aromas, especially when you associate particular aromas and blends with events in your life or specific emotions.

Indulge in the blends and aromas you love every day with the products you've created with these recipes, and with products you "invent" by incorporating your favorite oils. Now that you have the mechanics down and the safety standards in mind, you're free to get creative.

Finding Your Blend

Do you have an affinity for citrus oils like orange and lemon, or for resinous oils like myrrh? Research your favorite oils. You may be interested in discovering where those plants are grown and what the oils have in common. Essential oil research can take you on an international journey as you learn about oils from different continents and climates. You may end up inspired to travel and experience essential oil distillation in person!

As you start to think like an Aromatherapist, begin blending beyond the recipes you've discovered in this book. Start creating your own simple diffuser blends or lightly tweaking the recipes you use around the house.

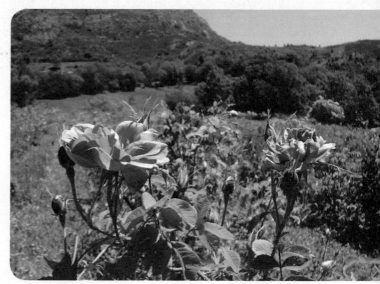

Add to your collection by buying oils in the categories you already love (such as conifers or floral oils), or by branching out to discover new oils.

If you're interested in learning more, you can start with Aromahead Institute's free online class, Introduction to Essential Oils (http://www.aromahead.com/courses/online/introduction-to-essential-oils). It's a great complement to this book, and a great way to establish a strong foundation in Aromatherapy.

It takes about 50 roses to make 1 drop of essential oil.

Appendix

Resources

Aromatherapy Certification Program

Aromahead Institute
www.aromahead.com

Andrea Butje
andrea@aromahead.com

Professional Organizations

The National Association for Holistic Aromatherapy
www.naha.org

Alliance of International Aromatherapists
www.alliance-aromatherapists.org

Bottles

SKS Bottle & Packaging, Inc.
www.sks-bottle.com

Purchasing Essential Oils and Carriers Online

1. Aromatics International
www.aromaticsinternational.com

Lolo, Montana. Aromatics International imports essential oils directly from distillers. Each batch of essential oil is GC or GC/MS tested. The GC report is on the website and can be printed. All the oils are either organic, wild crafted or un-sprayed. Also a great source for individual bottles, carrier oils, hydrosols, butters and diffusers.

Karen Williams,
karen@aromaticsinternational.com

2. Essential Elements
www.essentialelementssite.com

St Petersburg, Florida. Imports essential oils directly from distillers. Each batch of essential oil is GC or GC/MS tested. All the oils are either organic, wild crafted or unsprayed.

Minta Meyer, Terese Miller
essentail.elements@mac.com

3. Stillpoint Aromatics
www.stillpointaromatics.com

Sedona, Arizona. Imports high quality essential oils directly from distillers. Most oils are GC or GC/MS tested. All the oils are either organic, wild crafted or unsprayed.

Joy Musacchio, Cynthia Brownley
Info@stillpointaromatics.com

Master List of Essential Oils in This Book

Balsam Fir (*Abies balsamea*) – for cold and flu, cleansing

Bergamot Mint (*Mentha citrata*) – aches and pains, cooling

Black Spruce (*Picea mariana*) – for cold and flu, cleansing, aches and pains

Carrot Seed (*Daucus carota*) – skin nourishing

Cedarwood (*Juniperus virginiana*) – for cold and flu, relieves congestion

Cypress (*Cupressus sempervirens*) – deodorizing, calming, colds and flu

Elemi (*Canarium luzonicum*) – warming, cold and flu

Eucalyptus dives (*Eucalyptus dives*) – for reducing thick mucus from cold and flu

Eucalyptus globulus (*Eucalyptus globulus*) – for cold and flu, relieves headaches

Eucalyptus radiata (*Eucalyptus radiata*) – cleansing, relieves headaches

Eucalyptus citriodora (*Eucalyptus citriodora*) – bug repellant

Frankincense (*Boswellia carterii*) – calming, skin nourishing, relieves headaches

Geranium (*Pelargonium roseum x asperum*) – antifungal, deodorizing, skin nourishing

Ginger (*Zingiber officinale*) – aches and pains, warming, stomach soothing

Gingergrass (*Cymbopogon martini var. sofia*) – cleansing, for cold and flu, cooling

Grapefruit (*Citrus paradisi*) – disinfectant, deodorizing, cleansing, cooling

Ho Wood (*Cinnamomun camphora ct linalol*) – calming, aches and pains

Helichrysum italicum (*Helichrysum italicum*) – skin nourishing, healing for bruising, skin issues

Jasmine absolute (*Jasminum grandiflorum*) – skin nourishing

Juniper (*Juniperus communis*) – disinfectant, deodorizing, cleansing, for cold and flu, aches and pains, warming

Lavender (*Lavandula angustifolia*) – calming, disinfectant, deodorizing, cleansing

Lemon (*Citrus limon*) – disinfectant, deodorizing, cleansing, cooling, relieves headaches

Lemongrass (*Cymbopogon citratus*) – antifungal, cooling

Distilled Lime (*Citrus aurantifolia*) – deodorizing, disinfectant, cleansing, for cold and flu

Mandarin (*Citrus reticulata*) – disinfectant, deodorizing, cleansing, for cold and flu

Myrrh (*Commiphora myrrha*) – calming, skin nourishing, warming

Neroli (*Citrus aurantium var. amara*) – emotionally uplifting, skin nourishing

Norway Pine (*Pinus resinosa*) – for cold and flu, cleansing, aches and pains

Orange (*Citrus sinensis*) – deodorizing, disinfectant, cleansing

Palmarosa (*Cymbopogon martini var. motia*) - antifungal, skin nourishing

Patchouli (*Pogostemom cablin*) – calming, skin nourishing

Peppermint (*Mentha x piperita*) – anti-microbial, pain relieving, helpful for travel sickness

Petitgrain (*Bigarade*) (*Citrus aurantium var. amara*) – calming, deodorizing

Ravintsara (*Cinnamomum camphora ct 1,8 cineole*) – for cold and flu, cleansing

Roman Chamomile (*Chamaemelum nobile*) – calming, soothing for stomach, sleep

Rosemary ct. camphor (*Rosmarinus officinalis ct camphor*) – for cold and flu

Rosemary ct. verbenone (*Rosmarinus officinalis ct verbenone*) – for clearing thick mucus and skin care

Rose otto or absolute (*Rosa damascena*) – skin nourishing, cooling

Sandalwood (*Santalum album*) – calming, skin nourishing, cooling

Saro (*Cinnamosma fragrans*) – for colds and the flu, aches and pains

Siberian Fir (*Abies sibirica*) – disinfectant, deodorizing, cleaning, for colds and the flu

Spikenard (*Nardostachys jatamansi, Nardostachys grandiflora*) – calming, skin nourishing

Tea Tree (*Melaleuca alternifolia*) – disinfectant, antifungal, cleansing, for colds and the flu

Vetiver (*Vetiveria zizanoides*) – for boosting your immune system

White Pine (*Pinus strobus*) – disinfectant, cleansing, for colds and the flu

Ylang Ylang (*Cananga odorata*) – calming, sleep, skin nourishing

Master List of Carriers in This Book

Aloe vera gel

Avocado oil

Castile liquid soap

Cocoa butter

Coconut oil

Hydrosols (lavender, rose and sweetgrass)

Jojoba oil

Rose hip seed oil

Salt (pink Himalayan or sea salts are good possibilities)

Shea butter

Tamanu oil

Trauma oil (herbally infused oil containing Arnica, Calendula, and St. John's Wort)

Unscented, natural lotion

Vitamin E oil

The Author

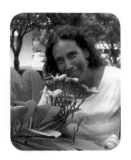

Andrea Butje
Aromatherapy Educator
Founder of Aromahead Institute

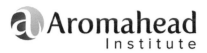

Since teaching her first Aromatherapy Certification Program in 1998, Andrea has developed the Aromahead Institute into a premier resource for Aromatherapy information and instruction. Today the Institute offers exclusive online educational resources including the scientifically based, 235-hour Aromatherapy Certification Program (approved by the National Association for Holistic Aromatherapy) and the Scholars Program, a 400-hour Program (approved by the Alliance of International Aromatherapists). Andrea utilizes the latest web tools to position the Aromahead Institute as a leader in online Aromatherapy education.

As a part of her commitment to high quality essential oils and education, Andrea travels internationally to work directly with distillers and small-scale organic farmers. She has visited and worked with distillers in Bulgaria, Canada, Corsica, Croatia, England, France, Greece, Italy, Morocco, Seychelles, Slovenia, South Africa, the United Arab Emirates, and the United States.

In 2004, she published the online International Directory of Essential Oil Distillers – a valuable resource database for those who want to import their own essential oils directly from organic, artisan distillers.

Andrea is changing the Aromatherapy educational paradigm through her inspired approach to teaching and creating community. Andrea creates and fosters online communities via Aromahead's monthly newsletter Essential News, Aromahead's blog, a Flickr account that highlights photographs from her visits to distillers, and an active Aromatherapy Facebook page. Aromahead Institute offers a graduate directory that highlights each student's work in the profession.

Andrea has also created several educational Aromatherapy videos that can be viewed on Aromahead's Youtube Video Channel.

Connect with Andrea through Aromahead Institute

- Online Classes at: www.aromahead.com

- Subscribe to Aromahead Weekly to receive a new Aromatherapy email each week. http:/www.aromahead.com/blog/ah-weekly-optin

- Blog: www.aromahead.com/blog

- Facebook: https://www.facebook.com/Aromatherapyeducation

Disclaimer

The information, content and product descriptions contained within this book are for reference purposes only and are not intended to and do not substitute advice given by a physician, pharmacist or other licensed health care professional. You may not use any of this information for treating a health problem or disease or to make a self-diagnosis. Information and statements in this book have not been evaluated by the FDA and are not intended to diagnose, treat, cure, or prevent any health condition or disease. If you have a medical issue you should contact your health care provider.

Notes:

Notes:

Made in the USA
Lexington, KY
28 September 2015